Hashimoto's Thyroiditis

The Sky's The Limit

A Daily Journal for Calming Coping Strategies

Rea Bachmann

Note: the suggestions in this book are not intended to replace a doctor's consultation.

CONTENTS

REA BACHMANN

ACKNOWLEDGMENTS

Thanks to: Nikki, Geli and Markus for their support.
The people I work with every day.
Hashimoto's Thyroiditis for being such a great teacher.

WELCOME

Dear reader,
welcome! I am very pleased you found your way here!

Were you diagnosed with Hashimoto's Thyroiditis? You are one of the many people who must learn to live with this thyroid autoimmune illness. Depending on the progress and the extent of the symptoms this can represent a great challenge.

As I have experienced Hashimoto's first hand for many years, I know virtually every symptom that can occur with this illness. I had to battle serious weight problems and concentration and memory deficiency, went through phases of deep depressive moods that were triggered by stress and diffuse anxiety and I had to deal with muscle and joint pains that appeared suddenly, moved and disappeared just as quickly.

At the same time I had the feeling I had lost myself and I no longer knew what my personality was. The world looked grey to me. And more importantly, I absolutely had no idea what was wrong with me before I was diagnosed.

I did not recognise myself any more. I had always been a positive person full of energy, with a lot of goals and the necessary strength to reach them.

Gradually I changed into an exhausted fighter who bravely battled on somehow, but without seeing the sense of it all. Whatever I tried - I always felt I functioned on 'empty batteries'.

It took many years before the illness was finally diagnosed by an attentive doctor. For me it proved positive to take both a traditional and an alternative medical route.

The urgently needed hormone substitution was done through traditional medicine. My thyroid glands were already that small because of the years-long infection that not taking that medication was unthinkable. I also had all the other hormonal regulation systems checked. Hashimoto's often also goes hand in hand with adrenal or sexual hormones imbalance. Please have these checked by a specialist if you feel that despite good medication your thyroid is not working better.

It took me a year to get wise, but I gradually felt better. Fluctuations were still on the daily agenda however and it took me a long time to get used to that roller coaster. I wondered what else I could do to improve my situation.

I wanted to find out more about my personal Hashimoto's and started a quest for clues. Why had my immune system turned against me? How had my past behaviour contributed to the situation and above all: how could I deal with it in future?

I was fully aware that no-one or nothing could give me back my ruined thyroid - but I wanted to do everything in my power to feel as healthy and productive as possible again.

Find out about alternative therapies near you and look at it as an opportunity to glance over the parapet and even benefit from your illness in the long term. Hashimoto's can be a good teacher that brings you valuable insights about yourself - if you feel like challenging yourself, going on a voyage of discovery and getting into it.

This day planner explicitly does not deal with the medical bases of Hashimoto's. There is enough literature about that. And tips for treatment and self-medication are now also readily available in the shops. I therefore want to pass on repetitions of that type.

This book follows another approach: What background issues can be found with Hashimoto's? Which exercises? Which self-reflection can you do to feel better? And how do you find the way back to what is really important to you?

Many people with thyroid problems shy away from openly expressing their wishes and needs. Often they are not even aware of them as they have learned to hold back over the years.

Fear often rears its ugly head too. Fear of rejection, fear of looking ridiculous, fear of loss and fear of living are but a few of the occurring types. Hashimoto's can be the incentive to start searching for your own, lost 'I'.

It can become a signpost on the way to start trusting your own inner voice again, to re-discover intuition and to find out with curiosity which opportunities the world still has to offer - if you dare to dream, to try and to listen to your soul.

The thyroid gland has the shape of a butterfly. I find that image very appropriate. With Hashimoto's, as a chronic infection, the immune system destroys the butterfly. It loses its wings, its lightness, spontaneity and elegance. Some butterflies remain in the phase before the metamorphosis, and stay in their cocoons as caterpillars - and miss out on the most beautiful things in life.

Hashimoto's can be a boost to re-conquer the butterfly qualities, to grow and to become aware of beauty and your own capabilities. You can control it yourself and target the backgrounds that pull you down, instead of being resigned to your fate of a chronic illness.

Every Hashimoto's illness is different. Some of the affected people swing back and forth between hyperthyroidism and hypothyroidism, some battle hot or cold nodes and others a goitre. The symptoms are different for everyone - but nevertheless we all have one thing in common: the wounded butterfly.

In this workbook we will address how to make your soul butterfly fly again. You will get an incentive on a specific theme every day. Of course you can decide for yourself how deep you want to go in those themes.

Hashimoto's illnesses are like a journey. We are never all at the same stage of the journey and sometimes we take shortcuts, because there is less to be learnt in those particular stages for ourselves than in others. This book does not pretend to be exhaustive. But it should give you incentives to explore your mental depths and give you a boost to find opportunities to make your life easier.

To me, Hashimoto's has now become a type of barometer. It clearly shows me when I have done too much, when I ignored limits, when I start working against myself and start living against my own priorities.

I am now often even grateful for it, because it stops me from putting myself in exhausting situations or to stay in negative situations for too long. Once you learn to view this illness as an inner guardian and to interpret its signals, it can be helpful.

I want to invite you on an exciting journey with this book. Possibly you will notice that many pieces of the jigsaw are falling into place. Maybe you will find ideas to lead your life in other directions and to become happier than you have been so far.

Hashimoto's should not be a curse - I see it as an opportunity. And I hope this book helps you to recognise the personal opportunities of an Hashimoto's illness. They exist. And they can give you a new perspective and light wings, once you discover them.

I wish you a pleasant and fulfilling journey to yourself.

Rea

REA BACHMANN

THE DAILY JOURNAL

As the title says, this is not advice, but a journal and workbook. Above all it's about personal reflection. I would like to inspire you and give you incentives every day to look deeper into your personality and the possible backgrounds of Hashimoto's, but above all into your goals and wishes.

They are still there despite a chronic illness and it is important to become aware of your strength that still exists at your core, despite all the exhaustion, fluctuations and many challenges.

How can you use this book optimally?

You will find incentives for every day that you can delve into as far as you want, and a few extensive topics too, that are dotted throughout the book as digressions. If a topic seems important to you you naturally will think about it more than about a topic that (currently) does not spark your need for information as strongly. Maybe it will get a new meaning later, that can change during the Hashimoto's journey. Therefore, just pick what seems important to you at the moment. You can't make mistakes when working with this book. Everything that happens leads you back to yourself a bit more.

In addition to stimuli you will also find a few questions about your condition. The daily targets are particularly close to my heart. Here you can write down what you have planned for the day (despite Hashimoto's - or rather because of it!). The point is not to do an awful lot, but to look at every new day in a positive frame of mind.

When you feel well you will of course plan to do a lot, but when you are having a bad day, you can plan less or simply allow yourself to 'rest'. Yes, that is allowed too!

Planning and writing down will help you to bring more structure back in your day-to-day life and at the same time to reflect on what you actually achieve despite a chronic illness. Most people don't realise how many challenges they overcome with flying colours every day.

By writing down your successes constantly, they will stay in your mind and you will value what you achieve. That's why there is a section at the end of every day where you can write down what you managed well, what you are proud of and what was important to you that day.

If you work with the pocket book version, you can simply write down your notes in your book. If you read the e-book, buy yourself a pretty notebook to write your daily notes in. Make sure that it is a notebook that you really like, because these notes are the turning and corner point for any change in your life with Hashimoto's.

It is important that you take them seriously. Initially you might find it senseless, or even ridiculous, to write down even little things - but great strength is hidden especially in these notes.

7

Therefore setting targets for every day is so important. It brings clarity to your life and makes it easier for you to progress.

You can often have the feeling you only run around in circles, endlessly. Usually that is not the reality. Something always moves forward. We only don't realise it, because we do not focus on it. This book should support you in leaving the hamster wheel and finding your way back to more ability to act and clarity.

Some people with Hashimoto's go through such severe phases of demoralisation that they hardly dare to go for goals. "I won't manage anyway", or "I don't have the energy" can often be heard.

Sorry, but I think that's an excuse. Every goal, however big, consists of many small stages. Those stages can be divided in tiny steps if necessary. And tiny steps are possible even with restrictive Hashimoto's! It is a matter of trust in yourself.

An example? OK...you got out of bed? Fantastic! Some don't even manage that! You motivated yourself for sport? Great! You ate healthily, you have informed yourself, you did not let others take advantage of you, you have not lived against your principles, you considered yourself important, you made someone laugh, you sorted out your clothes closet, cleaned the house, met up with friends, discovered a new hobby, went for a walk, completed a job well, daydreamed or finally sent a long planned postcard? Outstanding!

These are all small successes in your daily life! And every step you make towards a specific goal brings you closer to it.

Nothing is too small or too unimportant to write it down, if you want to get aware of your successes despite Hashimoto's. Don't shy away from writing down things that might seem ridiculous in comparison with other people. The point is not what others achieve. It is all about you.

ONLY ABOUT YOU.

Great, actually, isn't it? You can deal with what you find important, what concerns you in this book. Probably this was often overlooked in the past, wasn't it? You can work on yourself here and enjoy it, because everything is allowed and nothing is imposed.

Enjoy that time with yourself. Allow yourself to enjoy those daily successes. And please consider yourself important enough to write them down every day. At least 3 successes a day should find their way into this book. When you can think of more, excellent! Write everything down. You can read it back later and rightfully be proud of yourself.

Before we start our journey together, I would like to ask you to enter an official contract with yourself. It confirms that you will look after yourself and give your all to feel better during the time you work with this book.

Contract with yourself

I, _____, herewith conform that for the period

of _____ to _____ I will especially look after myself well and

do anything to feel better. I lovingly look after myself, listen to what my

body and mind need and enjoy the time I can spend with myself. I allow

myself nice things whenever I can and make sure that I have a wonderful

time. This contract cannot be terminated and can be extended after the end

of the above period at all times.

Place, date   Signature

REA BACHMANN

PLANNING OF THE FIRST WEEK

Welcome to the first week! We now start our mutual journey and firstly I would like to ask you that you generally reflect on what would be important for your future. What does the life you would like to have (despite or rather because) your Hashimoto's illness look like? How do you want to feel in the long term, who would you like to be, what would you like to achieve? What are your plans, your dreams, your wishes?

Please write down that goal here. It is important that you express it as if it was already a reality. I give you the example of the goal I set myself a few years ago when I started to look into Hashimoto's. At the time I felt bad physically and psychologically, but I didn't want to accept that this illness made my life so difficult.

I had to fight severe muscle and joint paints and excess weight and often only felt absolutely and utterly exhausted. But that was not how I wanted to spend the rest of my life. I therefore wrote down what popped up in my head instead:

I, Rea, live an active and happy life. My muscles and joints feel light and free and I have enough energy to do all that is important to me. I enjoy spending time with people I love and allow myself enough breaks alone with myself. I take the time I need, set boundaries when necessary, and enjoy every single day.

That is only an example of possible goals. It could be completely different topics for you. Express it as it feels comfortable to you. Important is: Write down what you WANT. Don't write down what you NO longer want.

I also could have written: I no longer have muscle pains. But that would have focused on the pain again. Instead I wanted light and free muscles - that I have today actually. The pain now only appears sporadically. And when it does, I know how to deal with it.

So: What do you wish from your life with Hashimoto's? I'm sure that after working with this book you will think of other goals, but for now just express what is currently important to you. You can change and adapt your goal any time. All this is a journey where you can also explore the little alleys left and right from the road, no strictly planned forced march. So: just go for it.

My goals

Before every week you will also find a short segment with a few questions on your plans for the coming days. Here you can enter what you are planning and what you would like to achieve. It could be about your health, your relationships, your job or other things that you hold dear. There are no limits.

How would you like to feel this week?

What would you like to achieve this week?

DAY 1 – LET'S GET STARTED

It's great you are here and we start together today! By working with this book and dealing with how your future journey with Hashimoto's can look like you take responsibility for your own life – and that is fantastic!

Many people take responsibility for anything and everything, worry about others and are always there when they are needed. The only thing they neglect is themselves, without even noticing it.

You are now going on a journey that will bring you back to yourself, back to your core, forward to your goals. I was always particularly interested in what is possible DESPITE and BECAUSE of Hashimoto's. Maybe your illness will make something possible that you would never have thought of otherwise? Could it even be that new doors open to you?

Hashimoto's thyroiditis really can be an opportunity. No-one can influence what life throws at us, but we can freely decide every day, every hour, every minute and every second with which mind-set and which behaviour we act on it. I wish you lots of wonderful Eureka moments! The only thing you need is some curiosity and the wish to fulfil yourself – even with a chronic illness.

How would you like to feel today?

What is important to you today? How would you like to plan this day?

Do you believe that some things are no longer possible with the illness? What are they? And why do you think that they cannot be part of your life anymore? Write down what you think of.

Please think about HOW you could still accomplish those things. What do you need for that?

Does something pop into your mind that you only discovered after your Hashimoto's diagnosis? What is it? And could many other things follow that you would not have encountered without Hashimoto's at all? Let those thoughts wander and write down the ideas that come to you.

Evening reflection

How did you feel today?

What have you achieved? What was fun? What are you proud of?

DAY 2 – HOW MUCH DO YOU KNOW?

It is important to be well informed about the symptoms and the treatment possibilities. Have you already looked into Hashimoto's? How well are you informed? Do you know which symptoms the illness triggers in you?

Hashimoto's is a "chameleon". It has many symptoms and that's why it is often not recognised correctly by doctors. Read about the illness. Inform yourself.

Reference books are better suited to internet forums in my opinion - for a simple reason: in forums people whose symptoms are usually severe share their experiences. They suffer great pain and that could give someone who has just started to look for information on the illness the impression that difficult symptoms are the rule. It does not have to be like that! It is very possible that your Hashimoto's is moderate, and that in the long run you will hardly notice the illness and be able to integrate it well in your life. So don't get worried.

Inform yourself about the illness and the possible treatments. That will also help you to be a lot more confident and relaxed in conversations with doctors and other therapists and to communicate your wishes for treatment a lot clearer.

What do you already know about Hashimoto's? Which of your symptoms do you attribute to the illness?

What would you still absolutely like to find out? How and where can you find the information to help you further?

How would you like to feel today?

What is important to you today? How would you like to plan this day?

Evening reflection

How did you feel today?

What did you achieve? What was fun? What are you proud of?

DAY 3 – DO YOU HAVE HASHIMOTO'S OR DOES HASHIMOTO'S HAVE YOU?

Yesterday the point was that you should be well informed. An auto-immune illness cannot be 'talked away'. But the question is how much you will let Hashimoto's define your life.

There is a thin line between 'being well informed' and 'becoming the hostage of an illness'. If you don't want Hashimoto's to define your whole life, you should make sure that you keep your progress (possibly modified) updated. It does not help you if you avoid any fun because you fear that your symptoms will worsen. Of course the exceptions are things that directly and negatively affect auto-immunity illnesses, such as e.g. excessive stress, smoking and the consumption of iodine.

I like to compare Hashimoto's to dancing on a tight rope. At the start you must cautiously put one foot in front of the other. And the more you get to know over time, the easier it gets. You find your balance again and here and there you can even dare a cheeky hop, because you know that you can master a brief balance loss. Allow yourself those hops in your life. Don't isolate yourself from everything that gives you pleasure. Your soul needs it.

In which areas of your life do you give the illness more room than is good for you?

How can you change that?

23

How would you like to feel today?

What is important to you today? How would you like to plan this day?

Evening reflection

How did you feel today?

What did you achieve? What was fun? What are you proud of?

SOURCES OF STRENGHT

Exhaustion, sometimes linked to nervous unrest, is very typical for Hashimoto's Thyroiditis. Suddenly everything seems too difficult, every road is too far away, every task too challenging. It is therefore really important that you find your own sources of strength and frequently tap into them.

Some people have never realised in their life that each of us needs resting points. Depending on how you have dealt with this issue until now, it could become a bigger or a smaller expedition.

Your own inner voice is a good compass here. Maybe you will have to learn to trust it again, but that is only a matter of practice. Preferably, ask yourself several times a day:

- **What do I feel now?**

- **How do I feel now?**

- **How does my body feel?**

- **How does my mind feel?**

- **Which thoughts do I have?**

- **Which challenges do concern me?**

- **What is surrounding me now?**

- **What would I PERSONALLY like now?**

The fact in itself that you ask yourself those questions and thus gently focus on your needs will already make a difference. You will increasingly get a feel for the things that harm and block you and what brings you back in balance.

Look at it as a game, that you can play completely 'unbridled'. There are no rules and you cannot do anything wrong. The point is only to be attentive and to establish what feels right or wrong to you at a given time.

Many people have lost that patience with themselves and the attentiveness to their own wishes in the daily hustle and bustle of life. Reclaim that ability. The questions listed above will bring you to your personal sources of strength where you can re-fuel.

DAY 4 – SETTING PRIORITIES

Even if you decide that the illness will not define your life - sometimes you have no strength at all with Hashimoto's. That is why it is even more important to set clear priorities.

Which tasks are really that important that they must be done immediately? In the case of an auto-immunity illness you have no strength to waste, and that makes it even more relevant that you can recognise time and energy intensive tasks that are not particularly urgent.

Hashimoto's patients are very often willing to go up to and beyond their personal limits. Everything must always be done perfectly and preferably immediately. But that thought cannot be achieved in every situation.

One of the tasks in living with Hashimoto's is to find your boundaries and to respect them. Important tasks of course require action and must be completed immediately - irrespective of how difficult it is. But because you free up capacities by setting less relevant tasks aside, you can dedicate yourself to the really important things - even when you have a bad day.

Who or what steals your time?

Who or what steals your energy?

In which areas can you delegate?

How can you become more efficient, without making more effort?

How would you like to feel today?

What is important to you today? How would you like to plan this day?

Evening reflection

How did you feel today?

What did you achieve? What was fun? What are you proud of?

DAY 5 - REMEMBER

Do you know when your Hashimoto's started? Can you link it to one particular event? Or did your symptoms gradually creep up on you, so you can't say for sure when they started?

Still, try to remember: Which decisive experiences occurred in your life? Which physical and/or emotional burdens were a great challenge to you? And what exactly made those experiences so difficult for you? Did you feel helpless? Not accepted? Overwhelmed? Or was it something completely different?

I want to emphasise that not every person with an auto-immune illness had a bad childhood or was the victim of violence. But there are many to whom this applies. That is why we are searching for traces in this book. Small jigsaw pieces can help you better understand yourself and deal with your illness in a different way. Write down in a table like this one what you think about.

Experience	Associated emotion

How would you like to feel today?

What is important to you today? How would you like to plan this day?

Evening reflection

How did you feel today?

What did you achieve? What was fun? What are you proud of?

DEPRESSIVE MOOD

Sometimes all the days are grey…

Badly controlled Hashimoto's can make your whole life a living hell. People who suffer from a thyroid illness are often actually pushed into the 'mental illness' corner. Of course there always is a link between body and mind - but as long as the hormonal system is not working properly, the best psychotherapy will not help.

If your medication is already optimal, melancholic phases and depressive moods can still happen. You are no different from everyone else on the planet. They are emotions that are part of us and that must be lived.

That can be very difficult because in such phases everything simply is too much for a person. Your nerves are frought and you don't understand that unfounded sadness that really 'takes you over'. Many people with those symptoms also withdraw from their circle of friends, because they can't even muster the strength for good experiences. The simplest of actions become almost impossible and high lethargy can lead to work, housework and even activities that usually make you happy are neglected.

Dealing with depressive episodes is a big challenge. If those melancholic phases increase, it is urgent to have another medical value check. Possibly something has shifted in the hormonal balance and the medication dosage must be adapted. Sometimes deficiency symptoms (vitamins, trace elements, anaemia) can trigger depressive moods. Please have them checked anyway.

If your medication is optimally adjusted and you still have down days you can see if the following exercise helps you:

In acute cases it was helpful for me to conscientiously withdraw, to concentrate on my breathing and to become fully aware of what is happening right now.

What do I feel? Sadness? Fear? Loss? Helplessness? Loneliness?

Examine which feeling motivates you and then ask yourself where it is noticeable in your body? Do you feel heavy pressure on your chest, a knot in your neck or a tightness in your heart? Do you feel pain in your belly, head or something else? How does the pain, the pressure, the tightness - or whatever you feel - feel exactly?

Localise which feeling is exactly where.

Once you get to the bottom of this you can try the next step: Visualisation - working with inner images.

It has always helped me to imagine, eyes closed, that instead of in the place taken over by the negative feeling, I was under a warm, golden sun. It brightens everything with its rays and dissolves the negative feeling progressively.

Experiment a little with this inner image. You can also place one or both hands on the affected place, to intensify your image.

It might look a bit strange to you to fight such heavy all-encompassing feelings with a visualisation - but this is a battle worth fighting!

Train yourself in letting this inner image become stronger and stronger. Do not give up. It can help you not feeling as lost, lonely and hopeless and bring you new energy.

DAY 6 – AWARENESS

Yesterday you have written down which experiences have heavily touched you in the past. Today I want to ask you to focus on *how* you mastered the challenges.

Which strategies did you use to get through that difficult time? Those abilities are still inside you - and now probably more refined and improved.

Could some of those also help with the difficulties you are faced with because of the Hashimoto's illness? Find at least three abilities that could currently help you. Become aware that you are ready for action!

The past problem	Past coping strategy	What could it be useful for today?

How would you like to feel today?

What is important to you today? How would you like to plan this day?

Evening reflection

How did you feel today?

What did you achieve? What was fun? What are you proud of?

LIFE PLAN

The thyroid gland also represents the expression of our personal life plan. These are our wishes, values and needs and how we achieve those.

Have you ever thought about your life plan? About everything that you want to achieve? What is important to you? What do you need to be truly happy? Grant ed, we only have one life - would it not be outrageous to use that precious time to the full and to enjoy it at the same time?

To get 'your money's worth' you need to know what makes you happy. You can find all this in your personal view of your life.

Your wishes

We all have very different wishes. The question behind this is: What do I really want? Mentally, psychologically, materially, in relationships, in the relationship with myself.

What are your true wishes? They are the incentive for everything you achieve day after day and can both encourage you and block you. It is therefore important, that you consciously think about what is really important to you.

What do you wish in your life? Write everything down. It can take up to 2-3 pages. Take all the space you need, and if necessary take an additional page if the space in this book is not enough. Write freely down what pops up in your head. It is important that you are honest to yourself. No-one except you will ever read this, unless you want them to. You don't have to hold back on anything or hide anything.

Your values

Do you know your values? Values are like inner programmes. They define what we consider right and good and act as a type of compass.

You cannot act against your values without becoming unhappy and feeling bad. An example: if fairness is one of your values, you cannot act unfairly without feeling pangs of conscience. If loyalty is one of your values you will not float with the tide without thinking and dump people once they have no more use. Etc... etc...

To find out what drives and blocks you it is important to know your values. Write down which value views you have. They influence your thoughts, your actions and therefore your whole life.

Values actually can change. Sometimes we have taken over values, e.g. from the family, that no longer make sense for us at present. Some long outlived values can become a real problem and stop you from being happy and lead a life as you imagine it. When you consciously reflect those blocks, you can start to let go of those old views and replace them with core values that are now important to you.

Take enough time and space for writing down these values too. It is important. What are your values?

Your needs

It is very simple: your needs tell you what you need to be happy. Basic needs like e.g. food, clothes, secure living accommodation, love, sexuality must be distinguished from other needs described as cultural or luxury needs. Those are about the need for cultural experience, consumption and the like. Luxury needs depend strongly on society and cannot be generalised.

Ask yourself which needs drive you. What do you miss? What would you like? What do you desire? Enclose both the basic and the cultural and luxury needs in this list.

Don't be afraid to write down what encourages you here. It is a very personal list. The notes of another person about this would definitely look completely different, but this is about you. So: let's write down those needs.

And? Have you dealt with these three questions? Very good! They are very important and affect your life not only in how you deal with Hashimoto's.

DAY 7 - PERFECTIONISM

Many people with auto-immune illnesses share a specific pattern: they are perfectionists and clearly expect more from themselves than from others.

At the same time they find it difficult to delegate responsibility.

Does that sound familiar to you? Be very attentive to the issue today. Whenever you notice that you lean towards perfectionism and you put yourself under unnecessary pressure, write the situation down in short. A few key words are enough.

It might sound weird, but: everything we become aware of and write down can be changed. It obtains another importance. You can better observe and classify your (exaggerated) demands to yourself - and you will be able to pull the brakes a lot quicker in future, because you are aware of the mechanisms. Which strategies can you use, to fall less into the perfectionism trap?

What would make you more relaxed?

Who can you trust, to whom can you delegate?

What makes your life easier?

How would you like to feel today?

What is important to you today? How would you like to plan this day?

Evening reflection

How did you feel today?

What did you achieve? What was fun? What are you proud of?

REA BACHMANN

OVERVIEW OF THE WEEK – WEEK ONE

Our first week together is over - time for a little review!

How did you feel in the past seven days? Did you find out new things or have you tried out new strategies? Did you have some thoughts you would like to examine more thoroughly?

Whatever you feel deserves more research, do it. It can lead you on important paths for you.

How did you feel in the past week?

What was important to you in the past week?

Which positive things have you achieved in the past week?

What was not that good yet in the past week? What would you like to improve?

PLANNING OF THE SECOND WEEK

Welcome to our second week together!

I think it's wonderful that you persevere and that you want to continue dealing with yourself. It shows that you take yourself seriously and that you are worth it to look after yourself.

What do you wish for your second week? What can you plan to live that week as fulfilled and happily as possible? Maybe you will already start to feel a bit listless just by looking at your day planner - many people hardly know how to deal with all the daunting challenges.

The fact that you keep going despite (or rather because of!) your Hashimoto's deserves respect and admiration. Allow yourself to be proud of yourself. It is not obvious that you get up every day and give it your best.

Once again: IT IS NOT OBVIOUS!

Which plans are you thinking of for this week?

How can you pamper yourself?

What is important to you this week?

DAY 8 – SELF-ESTEEM & SELF-LOVE

Perfectionist people are perfectionists for many reasons. A lack of self-esteem is often an important point. Perfectionism is generated from the fear of failure. Wanting to avoid errors at all costs, because you could be rejected or seen as incompetent - is an issue that can be found in many people with auto-immune conditions.

The feeling of being not worth much is rooted in childhood. Often - but of course not always! - thyroid patients come from families that showed them little recognition. That happened due to lack of understanding or attention, and often also simple ignorance and definitely not with bad intentions - but it gave the child the lasting impression that all its talents, interests and dreams are not worthy.

Many people with thyroid complaints are extremely sensitive. It is not hard to imagine the wounds the careless treatment of those sensitivities have caused already in childhood.

At some point the process became automatic. And now it is your own inner voice that always makes you doubt. There are cases where people actually hate themselves. The lack of self-esteem can lead to self-sabotage of various types. There is not enough self-confidence, not enough action, not enough fighting for the own dreams and visions. Or the exact opposite: They work to the point of exhaustion. And it never is good enough.

Occasionally eating disorders appear that make everything even more difficult. If you are unhappy with yourself and your image, you will find it very difficult to build up a positive self-image.

Many people concerned also have a great desire for harmony and serenity, which means they prefer to give in than to fight for their own convictions. It seems easier to remain low profile than to assert themselves - and risking criticism.

Do you recognise yourself in that description? Are you aware where exactly your self-esteem hit rock bottom? Write down your wounds today. Which thoughts and/or which behaviour triggers those recurring (destructive!) thoughts that you are worth very little?

There are endless possibilities to build up your self-worth piece by piece and to strengthen it. That is incredibly important, because with low self-esteem you live as if you were caged. But life as so much more to offer!

Please write down 5 things that you succeeded every day. Yes. Every day! You can link that to your work with this book and absolutely continue it after our time together is over.

Why? There is no easier and more effective way to realise what you achieve every day. You are worth to be noticed - above all by yourself! So be worth it to write down your successes. They can be little things. Maybe you made someone smile? Looked after yourself well? Exercised, ate healthy, relaxed, completed something important at work? Write it down every day. In the long term you will have a treasure chest full of achievements.

Once something is written down it gains another value. You absolutely should be worth it to yourself to write everything down. You will see, it will have a very positive effect.

How would you like to feel today?

What is important to you today? How would you like to plan this day?

Evening reflection

How did you feel today?

What did you achieve? What was fun? What are you proud of?

SMALL SELF ESTEEM EXERCISE

1) Draw a black stick figure. It represents you. It should not be a work of art, but make sure that you draw details too, such as eyes, mouth, fingers and feet.

2) Highlight everything you like about your body in green and everything you don't like in red. Turn the page and read again after you have completed this exercise.

And? Have you drawn your stick figure? How much is green, how much is red? Self-confident people tend to mark a lot in green, because they have a strong positive self-image. The lower the self-esteem, the more red parts will be shown in the drawing.

What does this exercise tell you about yourself and your subjective self-worth?

On which points can you work today to gain a better feeling for yourself and to strengthen you mentally in the long term?

WEIGHT PROBLEMS

I want to give inspiration for dealing with Hashimoto's in this day planner - but I also want to address the problems that I had to face in particular.

Weight was one of those challenges and the fact that I continued to gain even more weight over many years has made me very unhappy. As I know many other people experience the same, there is a special section about that theme in this book.

I don't know anyone with Hashimoto's - at least in the hypofunction phase - who has not experienced weight problems. And I don't know anyone for whom that does not represent a huge psychological and physical burden. Suddenly the weight increases almost uncontrollably even nothing has changed in the daily life. Most people affected by Hashimoto's eat extremely carefully and sensibly, practice sport, avoid alcohol - and despite all that the pounds are piling up.

The feeling of being helpless against that part of the illness often increases depressive moods. Higher body weight makes even more lethargic and life becomes a constant battle: against self-doubt, against weight, against tiredness, against the perceived lack of self-control, against yourself. Many Hashimoto's patients with weight problems hardly dare to leave the house out of fear of being ridiculed or despised because of the excess kilos. It is harder to find a good job, it is harder to deal with day-to-day problems with confidence, relationships and friendships suffer - ultimately it is more difficult to be happy. I suffered under this challenge more than once.

In the worst times I carried about 30 kilos of excess weight. When you are 162 cm tall and you weigh 89 kilos life simply is no fun anymore. You hardly dare to do anything, you avoid the outside world, you withdraw. That feeling dominated my whole life as a student. I ate healthily, exercised, but nothing changed. I had a vegetarian diet, hardly any fat and even took part in a weight loss clinic organised by the health service for many months - with the result that the scales showed even 7 kilos more than before. I developed a severe eating disorder, followed several therapies to get a grip on it, and despaired about my assumed lack of self-control. With hindsight this was pure torture - over many years.

When I was finally diagnosed with Hashimoto's I was almost 30 years old, had completed my degree and just started a new life in another city. With the medication 10 kilos disappeared in a short time - which was a miracle to me. My whole body seemed to breathe again and I only noticed then how exhausted I had been the whole time. I still fail to understand how I managed to stand my daily life with the double burden of studying and holding a student job for years.

My story is not exceptional, it is actually more the rule with Hashimoto's. It is therefore very important to me to emphasise this is NOT caused by a lack of self-control. If your medication is not appropriate you can stand on your head - you will not lose one gram.

In my case finely tuned hormone values helped a lot. I then experimented with various types of nutrition in the next years. I think that everyone must find out what works for them. I know Hashimoto's patients who thrive on vegan food (without soy of course). It absolutely did not work for me. I did not lose weight and my health was not great.

I lived on a strictly raw diet for a while and felt really well - but the weight hardly changed. What helped me finally to control my weight problem, to continue losing weight and feeling really well, was the transition to ketogenic nutrition, e.g. Paleo. Maybe you feel like informing yourself about this topic, it would go beyond the context of this book - and is many worth a new book...

The most significant change had to take place in my head. From the start of the weight problem, it had been pumped into my head from all sides that fat is the root of all evil and must be avoided at all costs. Instead I was supposed to eat lots of carbohydrates - brown bread, whole-wheat pasta, all sorts of cereals. And of course vegetables and fruit.

As I know now that was a catastrophe for me especially. Not only am I wheat intolerant and it causes stomach pain and worsens the muscle cramps - I also was constantly hungry, my blood sugar levels were like a yo-yo and over the years I developed a stubborn insulin resistance and increased cholesterol levels. If I had continued like that I would inevitably slid into Type 2 diabetes.

My last desperate attempt was the absolute opposite of everything that is commonly recommended. I excluded all the wheat products, potatoes and rice from my diet, and ate lots of fish, meat and eggs, huge quantities of vegetables and fruit from time to time. I reduced dairy products as much as possible. A large part of my energy comes from fat - yes you read it right: fat! Butter, cream, oils (coconut oil in particular), nuts and seeds.

Low Carb High Fat has proven to be my salvation and is clearly the type of nutrition that suits my body best. And my mind too. Cravings are a thing of the past and sweet food just no longer interests me. I feel great, the insulin resistance is decreasing and my cholesterol levels are lower than ever. And I keep losing weight. Today I only have 8 more kilos to lose to reach my normal weight and for the first time, since living with Hashimoto's, I feel the illness no longer controls me.

That was my journey, as I said before. Maybe it could be an incentive for you. Maybe your way out from the kilo trap is completely different, because your body works differently and needs something else - it's possible!

I would simply like to warmly invite you not to exclude anything offhand. Don't be bullied into anything that does not suit you or your body. Watch out for yourself, get all possible information you can get, share experiences with other people concerned. There are many ways to Rome. Find the path that is easy and free to you.

Weight can be a protection... Do you need a "thick skin" or did you need one in the past? Is that still the case today?

What would be different in your life if you were slim?

What can you do to start on the road to a healthy and suitable weight? Which information do you need? Who or what can support you?

DAY 9 - CHILDHOOD

What do you spontaneously think of when you think of your childhood? Which images do you see in your head? What was your childhood like, which smells do you remember, which colours, which feelings, which sounds? Were you happy? When? And were there times you were sad? If so, why?

Many auto-immune patients were already in a situation where they had to mediate a lot as children and had little room for themselves. Maybe you had to be very "adult" as a child. Maybe you had no real opportunity to live out your childhood dreams or you felt "wrong" at the time already.

Look at your childhood today. It is important that you don't have to force anything. Just curiously delve into your memories. What comes to mind and what are the feelings associated to them? Which childhood dream can your adult self achieve today?

Write a letter to your 9 year-old self. What would you like to tell that child? What do you consider important from your current perspective? What should you as a child pay attention to? What should you fight for? What do you give for the journey?

How would you like to feel today?

What is important to you today? How would you like to plan this day?

Evening reflection

How did you feel today?

What did you achieve? What was fun? What are you proud of?

DAY 10 - FAMILY

What do you associate to the word 'family'?

Positive? Negative? Sometimes it is useful to differentiate between the biological family we originate from and the people we have now created or would like to create our own family with.

Nobody can chose their biological family. We are born into specific structures and must deal with them - whether we like it or not. That biological family has given you many things for your life journey and the question is whether you find this important or not - and above all, whether you allow that unpleasant childhood experiences still slow you down today.

We have no power over the challenges life will set us. But we do have an influence on the way we are dealing with old patterns. If something that deeply hurt you as a child still prevents you from freely acting according to your personality, you have the right of letting it go in full awareness today. That does not 'undo' anything, but you can decide not to give the old ghosts the power over your current strength, life and happiness.

Which issues from your childhood are you at war with?

Do these inner fights give or take energy?

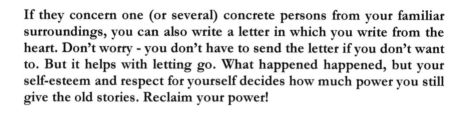

If they concern one (or several) concrete persons from your familiar surroundings, you can also write a letter in which you write from the heart. Don't worry - you don't have to send the letter if you don't want to. But it helps with letting go. What happened happened, but your self-esteem and respect for yourself decides how much power you still give the old stories. Reclaim your power!

How would you like to feel today?

What is important to you today? How would you like to plan this day?

Evening reflection

How did you feel today?

What did you achieve? What was fun? What are you proud of?

REMORSE

Many people continue to feel remorse, but it is rarely admitted or spoken about. But the unpleasant feeling can hang over us like a dark cloud forever. Whether the remorse is linked to a family experience, relationships or work - we are not free in our decisions and actions if we have not processed old events and keep punishing ourselves.

Some issues cannot (any longer) be resolved - which makes it even more important to forgive yourself and to integrate the old experience as valuable in the here and now. Also: most people regret much more what they haven't done than mistakes at the end of their lives. There are things in life we dream of and that we daren't 'go for' - for whatever reason - and that we will regret later. Interesting, isn't it?

If remorse is one of your issues, you can explore it further with the following questions.

What do I regret?

Why do I regret it?

What should I have done differently to not feel regret today?

Is there something I can do to turn the past mistakes or past omission around ? What?

For what do I condemn myself?

How hard do I judge others? How hard do I judge myself?

Which facades do I keep up?

For what could regret be good in my case?

How can I transform regret into something useful?

How good am I at forgiving myself? What can I do to forgive myself?

What do I have to forgive others for to find peace of mind?

DAY 11 – SELF-EXPRESSION

In alternative medicine the thyroid corresponds to throat chakra. Its colour is sky blue, and the associated themes are self-expression, truth, communication, integrity and authenticity and the connection to the higher self.

This leads us to interesting questions, such as: How authentic are you? How strongly do you live your own inner personality? How often and clearly do you communicate? Can you express what moves you? In every life situation? In every conflict?

To live your life to the full you need the courage to show yourself, to take positions and to be seen as authentic and an individual. Have you already realised how unique you are on this planet? No-one else is like you! And no-one can achieve things the same way as you...

Quite impressive don't you think? There is only one you, once. The world deserves that you show yourself with everything you are, can do and know. How you do it, the path you chose of course is up to you.

How do you currently express your personality?

What would happen if you immediately let your inner light shine out? How does your environment react? What would improve, what would possibly be worse than before?

How would it benefit you if you allow yourself to fully be yourself and show your individuality with confidence?

It can take courage to assert yourself authentically and clearly. What are you afraid of?

What exactly can you do today to express yourself? How can you be open and centered in your needs? In which area of your life should that expression take place?

How would you like to feel today?

What is important to you today? How would you like to plan this day?

Evening reflection

How did you feel today?

What did you achieve? What was fun? What are you proud of?

DAY 12 – WORK

What does work mean to you? Are you happy with what you do? Can you function without excessively exhausting yourself, do you take enough breaks, does your work fill you with pride, contentment and sense?

I think that we can only be really good in things that are really close to our hearts. And even more radically I think that it is a waste of a precious life to work in a job that does not truly fulfill us. Maybe Hashimoto's disease is an indication for you that also tests your current work situation.

For me personally the illness made it very importantly clear to me that I must not do everything. Nor endure everything. Nor participate in everything and tolerate and above all excuse everything. I *must not do* anything - but I am *allowed* to do anything.

I have consciously decided to change the circumstances in my life. It was impossible to continue the way it was, sooner or later the health price I would have had to pay would have been too high - not to mention the effects on my mind. Starting and continuing all those changes was not easy and it took a while before everything fell into place. But the result has been worth it.

Like a big jigsaw, the pieces gradually formed a new, much more coherent picture for me. Today I love my work. I am free to plan my time as I please and I can react to the progress of my Hashimoto's flexibly if it is necessary. If you now think: "Good for you, but that's impossible in my work!" I would like to give you a few incentives:

How can you adjust your environment in such a way that your working life becomes fulfilling and happy? Often you underestimate what can be changed!

Write down the keywords that are important to you. How could you work efficiently and feel good at the same time? What do you need to be very productive?

If your current work does not allow flexibility - who says that you actually have to stay in that job? Think of the opportunities you could grasp if nothing could go wrong. What would you do then?

Which ideas that you have written down can be achieved in reality? Maybe it takes some effort ... Or courage... Or a radical change of thought patterns. But what is so dear to you that it deserves a real chance?

Find an action today that makes your working life easier and more fulfilling and really implement it. No compromises.

How would you like to feel today?

What is important to you today? How would you like to plan this day?

Evening reflection

How did you feel today?

What did you achieve? What was fun? What are you proud of?

DAY 13 – FREEDOM

Empowerment, autonomy and freedom are other themes associated with the thyroid and the throat chakra.

Many Hashimoto's patients tend to hide their light under a bushel. They find it hard to imagine how to act self-confidently and independently - mostly out of fear of hurting other people or to stand out unpleasantly.

In which areas of your life do you desire more freedom?

How does that freedom look to you? How can you provide it to yourself in future?

What is the worst that could happen if you claim your freedom, independence and empowerment?

What is the best that could happen to you when you do?

Find an action that strengthens your freedom, independence and empowerment today and apply it. Irrespective of what others think about you. What do you decide?

How would you like to feel today?

What is important to you today? How would you like to plan this day?

Evening reflection

How did you feel today?

What did you achieve? What was fun? What are you proud of?

DAY 14 – SELF-EFFICIENCY

Many Hashimoto's patients complain about feeling helpless and powerless. They are tired and without energy for anything. If your medication is not optimal yet, don't get put off or fobbed off. Please demand that everything is thoroughly tested.

Maybe a T4 mono drug is not enough. Maybe you suffer from a transition dysfunction. Possibly the iron levels are not optimal or there is a lack of vitamin D or vitamin B12.

There are endless reasons why you are tired and exhausted. Be stubborn, read up about your illness (there are many good books on the market now) and stand up for yourself. You can evaluate best how you feel - and as long as your situation is not satisfactory, please stay on the ball.

Self-efficiency means that we make things happen and assert what is important to us. The fact that you will not be treated like a toy - at work, in the family or at the doctor's - will strengthen your feeling of self-worth in the long term.

Use every opportunity now to make yourself important. Of course you should not become an egocentric monster - a fear many people with thyroid complaints have as soon as they start to set boundaries and implement them. But that fear is mostly unfounded. You will not become self-centered only because you consider yourself important. On the contrary. You only increase the (long overdue!) perception of your own worth. It will do you good.

What can you do today to be self-efficient? Where can you move something that is important to you?

How would you like to feel today?

What is important to you today? How would you like to plan this day?

Evening reflection

How did you feel today?

What did you achieve? What was fun? What are you proud of?

OVERVIEW OF THE WEEK – WEEK TWO

Another week is behind you. You surely have tried out and written down a lot - and you can be proud of yourself because you stay on the ball! A summary can help to become aware of the point you're at, what is done and what is still in motion.

How did you feel in the past week?

What was important to you in the past week?

Which positive things have you achieved in the past week?

What was not that good yet in the past week? What would you like to improve?

PLANNING OF THE THIRD WEEK

Hello and welcome to our third week together!

How are you? What is your outlook for the next seven days? Here you will find room to establish what is important to you, what you would like to achieve, and what you particularly want to pay attention to.

A week can be lived with much more clarity and serenity, if we are aware of what we expect from ourselves and others. Take the time to take notes.

How would you like to feel this week?

What would you like to achieve this week?

DAY 15 - CREATIVITY

Self-expression of course is part of creativity. There are so many fields creative expression is possible in. You can write, cook, work in the garden, crafts, paint, draw or sing, learn to play an instrument, design furniture or clothes ... the possibilities are virtually endless.

It helps many Hashimoto's patients to deal with the illness and the associated burdens in a creative way. There is a way to express yourself and also to let the unconscious level influence. You don't have to explain anything generated in the creative process. You also should not try to be especially "good". Everything originates from within you and precisely therefore it is important how it actually is.

Hashimoto's is quite similar to a butterfly coming out of its cocoon. As long as you do not live your self-expression - in any area - freely, you are like a caterpillar in a cocoon. The cocoon protects but also limits movement. You only can decide whether you want to discover and express the individuality inside you. Creativity can be a wonderful first step on that journey. Grab the opportunity! It can only be beneficial.

Where can you become creative? Find an area that you enjoy. It is not about perfectionism. It is about freely releasing what is waiting to be expressed inside you.

Start today with a little creative work. A short poem? A sketch? A wild colourful painting? A new recipe invented by you? A song? Whatever appears, give it room. Self-expression lets you fly in this world. Allow yourself to show yourself.

How would you like to feel today?

What is important to you today? How would you like to plan this day?

Evening reflection

How did you feel today?

What did you achieve? What was fun? What are you proud of?

DAY 16 – REST & BREAKS

The daily life of most people is dominated by stress and performance. There always is something to do, life becomes increasingly faster and the tasks to achieve are increasingly complex.

How much rest do you allow yourself? And how many breaks do you take? Do you force yourself to have some time off from all the daily activity or do you celebrate it? Can you switch off your smartphone from time to time? Are you still capable of enduring tranquillity or do you find it hard?

It is not always easy to take the rest you need. Auto-immune processes will force us at one point to do so, if we do not recognise the signals our body gives us on time.

How do you notice early exhaustion in yourself?

What are your resources to 'reload'? What gives you energy? Remember the questions about the sources of strength.

How do you deal with your need for rest? Are you ashamed you need breaks? If so, why?

Can you come to rest? Without distraction? How is that for you?

In which areas are you too quiet? Where do you lack zest for life, enthusiasm? Where do you stop?

How would it be if you set a few small conscious breaks in your daily life? Five or ten minutes are often enough to switch off and to think of something else. Use memory aids to make sure you don't exceed your rest times, e.g. the alarm on your mobile. You will notice that you go back to your work a lot more focused after a short conscious relaxation time.

Which memory aids can you use?

Is your environment involved? Can you rely on understanding? If not - set clear boundaries. No-one can evaluate your need for rest as well as you! And no-one has the right to tell you if and when you can rest.

Of course compromises are always necessary. But it is important that you learn to consider yourself important at this level too. You are entitled to rest and to time to collect yourself. Take it and above all: take it without feeling guilty. Your body and mind will thank you for it.

How would you like to feel today?

What is important to you today? How would you like to plan this day?

Evening reflection

How did you feel today?

What did you achieve? What was fun? What are you proud of?

FEAR

Many people with thyroid dysfunctions know fear. It often is linked to signs of depressive moods and in severe cases can lead to panic attacks. If you suffer from panic attacks please seek professional therapeutic support. This book is not enough in that case. As I assume that you take the responsibility for yourself and your health - otherwise you would not be reading this book - I count on your understanding.

For all others who wonder why they keep having to face diverse paralysing anxious feelings, I have listed a few questions here that could shed some light on things.

What am I scared of? Is the fear diffuse or can I precisely name what makes me fearful?

What stifles me?

How do I deal with criticism?

How do I deal with conflict and arguments?

Can I stick to my guns? In which situations do I find it easy and when do I find it hard?

What should I learn, to be more confident?

How do I deal with insecure life conditions?

How do I show myself to the world and my surroundings?

How do I stage myself and when do I show my true self? Who is allowed to meet my true self? Why?

Can I let control go or do I find it quite difficult?

To which extent do I trust myself?

Do I dare to experiment even if I don't know where it might lead? In which cases can I do that? When is it difficult?

How spontaneous am I? What stops my spontaneity from flowing freely?

Fears are often linked to low self-esteem, with a strong need for security and little trust in the own ability of being able to deal with difficult situations too. Please remember difficult and/or fear-inducing moments in your life and remember the strategies that helped you at the time. They can be very useful now too.

DAY 17 – SELF-SACRIFICE

Do you tend to always give everything for others and to sacrifice yourself? Even when you notice that you get little or no thanks for that? Welcome to the club - many people with auto immune illnesses experience the same.

It is obvious to them always to think about the well-being of others first and to take the back seat. Some get the feeling at some point to actually be completely 'invisible' with their own wishes and needs and to be constantly overlooked. That can be desirable when the feeling of self-worth is so low that you would actually prefer not to be noticed at all. But of course you can't really enjoy life like that.

Hashimoto's Thyroiditis sets an important task: setting boundaries. It is all about showing boundaries to others that should not be crossed ('Up to here and no further!') and keeping to your own boundaries.

If you tend to always do too much, to work too hard, to give too much, you permanently cross the healthy boundaries of your personality.

You cannot keep demanding that much from yourself without burning out. It is therefore important to be aware of how you deal with boundaries.

In which areas do you tend to sacrifice yourself? How does that feel?

How do you deal with boundaries and setting boundaries? Which feelings crop up when you think about it?

Can you set clear boundaries if someone demands something from you that you actually are not willing to give? Or do you transgress that inner obstacle to please others? If you do, why? What are you afraid of?

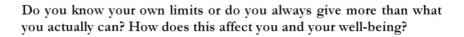

Do you know your own limits or do you always give more than what you actually can? How does this affect you and your well-being?

What would happen if you accept your limits and lovingly integrate them in your life? The point is not to forbid yourself something. It is to gain more strength, because you stop feeding things that suck up your energy.

Do you take enough time for yourself? If not, start doing so. Give yourself time off that you spend with yourself alone and fill that time with things that make you feel good and make you stronger.

Music? Sport? A long walk? Reading? Shopping? Whatever you enjoy set enough time aside for it.

How would you like to feel today?

What is important to you today? How would you like to plan this day?

Evening reflection

How did you feel today?

What did you achieve? What was fun? What are you proud of?

RELAPSE INTO OLD PATTERNS

While you are working on yourself, there will come a time, sooner or later, when you will think everything is collapsing inside you again. Old behaviour patterns and belief systems are stubborn. But what is a relapse actually? Nothing more than a short term step on grounds that have been familiar to you for a long time and therefore feel more secure than the lightness of the butterfly that still flies slightly erratic and insecure in the air.

When you notice that you are sliding back into old thought patterns or behaviour - no panic! Breathe. Relax. A short stopover will not stop you from soaring high again. You only have to consciously decide it.

Every day you have the absolute free choice which thoughts and behaviour you choose. You can decide the extent that something sets you off course. As I said before - you cannot influence the cards you are dealt in life. But you always have the choice how to react to them, whether you let them block you and strike you down, or whether you remain consciously balanced - or find your way back to that after a short breather. Because you want it.

Don't let throwbacks drive you crazy, they are simply part of it. Anything else would not be human. Consider them as a part of the road and continue your journey. Ultimately, it always brings you back to yourself - and you alone define the pace of your journey. No-one can and will do it for you and that precisely is a wonderful and big chance to shape your life as you want it - Hashimoto's or not.

Emergency aids for relapses

* Write messages to yourself! Use post-its or little notes where you write down why you have decided in favour of more lightness, freedom and self-expression. Stick those messages on the bathroom mirror, the fridge or another place that you see often. They will keep reminding that this journey is worth it. That will keep you on track on difficult days.

* Find a song that symbolises that positive journey to yourself for you. A song that you associate with self-confidence, independence, authenticity and strength. Listen to it when you feel bad. It will help you reflect again on the essential - your own strength and inner light that wants to be lived.

* You can also choose an object to remind you and carry it with you always. A pretty stone e.g., that you can carry in your pocket as your "rock in the storm". Or something else, that you can hold and that reminds you how valuable you are and the strength that lives inside you. My 'anchor' is a pretty small gold coin.

* Scents are precious anchors too, that you can associate with strength, self-worth and freedom. Choose a scent you like, e.g. an essential citrus oil or lavender, rosemary or orange - whatever feels right to you. On days when you are plagued by doubts or you relapse into old patterns, a few drops on a handkerchief or in a diffuser can help. The scent will help you to focus on your goals again.

* Awareness can also be a great support. Especially on difficult days it is important that you are aware of positive things. For example you can tell yourself how nice it is when you feel the sun shine on your nose. Or how nice it is that you can go for a walk in the fresh air. Or how nice it is to enjoy tranquillity while you lay in bed. Or how nice it is that you smell the flowers in a florist's on the way to the train station. Small things that deserve to be noticed.

The point is absolutely not to tell yourself that everything is wonderful and to superficially suppress the bad things. It is much more about consciously experiencing moments and being in the here and now. If your attention wanders to something nice, there is no room for negativity in that time slot. That basic attitude can make a bad day easier for you.

DAY 18 – GIVE & TAKE

Giving and taking must be balanced for real contentment to be achieved. Hashimoto's patients often tend to give relentlessly and to suppress their own needs. Taking or accepting is very difficult for them on the contrary. In the long term that leads to dissatisfaction and self-resentment.

In which situations do you find it easy to give? When is it difficult?

In which areas of your life do you find it easy to take? When is it difficult?

Where could you consciously decide to take as much as you give in future in a specific area of your life?

What would happen if you suddenly only would give half? What would be the worst that could happen? And the best?

How would you like to feel today?

What is important to you today? How would you like to plan this day?

Evening reflection

How did you feel today?

What did you achieve? What was fun? What are you proud of?

DAY 19 – SELF-DESTRUCTION

Auto immune illnesses are processes in which the immune system turns against the body's own structures. It aggressively works against your own body. That is also the case with Hashimoto's thyroidism. Various factors are considered as origins. Viral infections, genetic predisposition, stress, nutritional defects, hormonal shifts - there is no certainty.

The question asked about self-destructive processes from an alternative medical perspective is: What led the immune system to suddenly turn against the person itself? The idea of self-destruction in a psycho-somatic context does not please everybody and some people would rather not deal with it. That is fine. It should not apply to everyone. If you are generally interested in this however, you will find a few questions below that can help you with your research.

Do you tend to 'swallow' a lot instead of expressing what displeases you?

Can you remember when it started? Was there a key experience, a trigger?

Why can't you deal with aggressions outwardly? What is stopping you?

Who has taught you that is not respectable? And above all: Would you like that person to still have power on your life today?

What would happen in the worst case scenario if you direct aggressions outwardly instead of against you? (Of course that does not mean that you should become violent against people, animals or objects. But it can mean e.g. that you communicate clearly and openly, when something displeases you. Do you remember? The throat chakra is linked to clear expression and communication!)

Which outlets for release of aggression do you spontaneously think of?

How would you like to feel today?

What is important to you today? How would you like to plan this day?

Evening reflection

How did you feel today?

What did you achieve? What was fun? What are you proud of?

DAY 20 – GOALS AND VISIONS

Hashimoto's can sometimes be so tiresome that you hardly dare to plan anything. At the end of the day you never know how you will feel the next day, the next week, in summer or next year. That can stop many people from making their dreams a reality.

Waiting behaviour leads to more stagnation however, and that can become frustrating. Nothing really moves anymore - everything secretly is always defined by Hashimoto's.

We dealt with your goals at the beginning of the book already, do you remember? You addressed how you would like to live despite a chronic illness. Let's get back to that.

It is very important that you have dreams, achieve your goals and develop long term visions. Hashimoto's or not, you deserve to live the life you desire and that makes you happy! Consciously decide today, that this illness will no longer stop you from working on making your dreams a reality. Maybe something has already changed in you during the work with this book. Therefore please address that theme again today.

What are your dreams? What would you like to achieve in your life?

Make at least one dream a concrete goal. That means that you clearly formulate WHAT you would like, HOW it makes you feel and WHEN you would like to achieve it. Do you remember how to express goals? The present tense is important. E.g. if you wish to open your own cafe, a possible goal expression would be:

"I [your name] operate from [insert date] a profitable and successful cafe in [insert place] with [insert number] employees. My work makes me happy, because I am my own boss".

Which dream do you turn into a goal today? Maybe you want to reach your ideal weight, go on a world trip, start a family or get your dream job? Don't let it just be a dream. Write down the goal and plan the steps required to achieve it. An Hashimoto's illness can sometimes change our priorities, but should never stop us from working on making our dreams a reality.

If you find it hard to set goals: imagine you are 90 years old and you are sitting in your rocking chair on the porch. What should the life you are reflecting on look like? Write it from the perspective of that 90 year-old!

How would you like to feel today?

What is important to you today? How would you like to plan this day?

Evening reflection

How did you feel today?

What did you achieve? What was fun? What are you proud of?

DAY 21 - OUTLOOKS

We have reached the last day of this book. You have intensively dealt with yourself in the past three weeks. How can it go further now?

I would suggest that you continue to writing down in short how you feel every day. It is important to write down positive experiences and of course the progress you notice. Write down at least five things every day that you succeeded - even if they are tiny. That way you direct the attention more to the successes in your life. That will make more stable in the long run and help you to better deal with throwbacks too. They will then not get you off course as easily.

You should also think which plans you have for the near future, what is important to you and how you want to spend the next months. Here are a few questions for this.

Which goals do you have for the next 3 months?

What is the main thing you should deal with now? What is important to you?

Which role can your Hashimoto's illness play in that timespan?

What will make your inner butterfly fly? What are you dreaming of? What can you do today to work on achieving it?

How would you like to feel today?

What is important to you today? How would you like to plan this day?

Evening reflection

How did you feel today?

What did you achieve? What was fun? What are you proud of?

OVERVIEW OF THE WEEK – WEEK THREE

Our last week together is behind you. How did it go? Did you manage to unlock new themes, made curious discoveries, experimented? Take your time to look back on the past seven days and make notes.

How did you feel in the past week?

What was important to you in the past week?

Which positive things have you achieved in the past week?

What was not that good yet in the past week? What would you like to improve?

AND NOW?

This is it - we reached the end of our journey together!

I hope you had fun with this book, you could take new ideas on board and you received many incentives for self-reflection. But above all, I hope that Hashimoto's will be a support instead of an obstacle for you in future.

Ultimately you decide how much influence you want to allocate that illness on your life. Of course you will encounter phases when things are not as smooth. It is important that you see those for what they are: nothing more than phases. You are not a machine. Fluctuations are normal! But you can immediately interpret them otherwise.

You can see the opportunities and positive challenges in them, instead of destructive obstacles. You can always get back up and work on your authenticity, self-expression, independence and freedom.

You have the free choice every day to decide to let the butterfly fly in lightness. The recognition in itself that you can choose should give you courage and confidence.

No-one forces you to fly euphorically always. You can be down for a day or longer from time to time. But you should realise that Hashimoto's does not prevent you from flying. Because you will not allow it.

The Sky's The Limit ... I wish you a wonderful life journey!

Rea

ABOUT THE AUTHOR

Rea Bachmann has been living with Hashimoto's for almost two decades and has experienced almost every symptom in person. She was already interested early on in the role of the mind in connection with the illness and what everyone can contribute to feeling better in themselves. Today Rea Bachmann supports Hashimoto's patients with complementary therapy to medical treatment.

MORE BOOKS FROM REA BACHMANN

Rea Bachmann is living in Berlin, Germany, so her books are usually published in German.

Hashimoto als Chance. Ein Arbeitsbuch. (This is the german version of "The Sky's the limit"). Rea Bachmann, 2015. Print and ebook.

Herausforderung Haut. Selbsthilfe bei Neurodermitis, Psoriasis und Co. Rea Bachmann, 2015. Print and ebook.

Thank you very much for reading *The Sky's The Limit*! Gaining exposure as an independent author relies mostly on word-of-mouth, so if you have the time and inclination, please consider leaving a short review on Amazon.

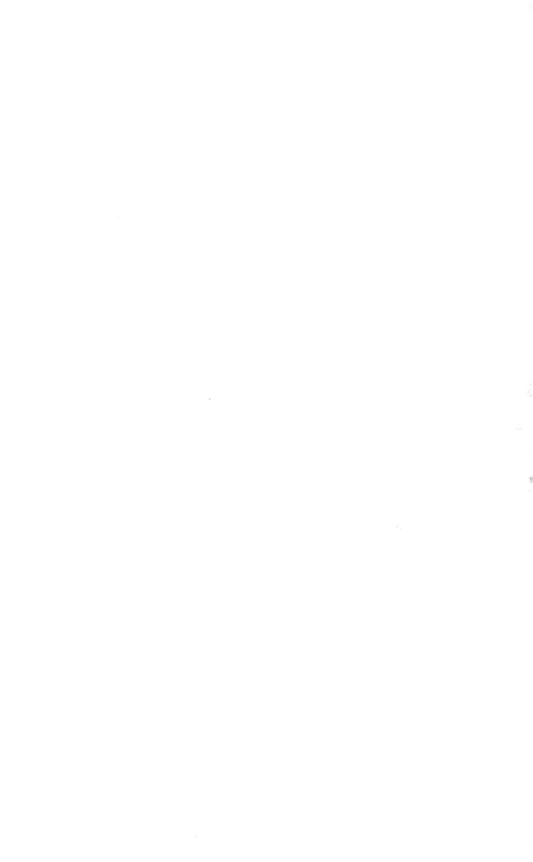

87743159R00093

Made in the USA
Lexington, KY
29 April 2018